Mastering Lucid Dreaming: Techniques to Unlock Your Inner Dreamer and Transform Your Life

Violet Payne

Preface

Dear Reader,

From as early as I can remember, I have been a lucid dreamer. My earliest memories are filled with vivid dreams where I had full awareness and control, transforming ordinary sleep into an extraordinary adventure. Growing up, I didn't realize that this ability was anything unusual or remarkable; it was simply a part of my nightly routine.

As a child, I often felt a lack of control over my waking life. Various circumstances made me feel powerless and overwhelmed. The one place where I found solace and empowerment was in my dreams. Here, I could escape the nightmares that plagued my sleep and create worlds where I had the ultimate control. This natural transition into lucid dreaming became a crucial coping mechanism during those challenging times.

Lucid dreaming allowed me to navigate through and conquer fears, turning horrifying nightmares into adventures and transforming distress into exploration. This powerful tool became a sanctuary, a place where I could not only escape but also heal and grow.

My understanding of lucid dreaming deepened significantly during my first year of undergrad. In one of my courses, a professor dismissively claimed that lucid dreaming was merely a hypothetical concept with no real basis. A student had inquired about the phenomenon, only to be met with skepticism. After class, I approached the student, eager to share my experience and reassure them of the reality and potential of lucid dreaming. I offered tips and techniques, many of which you will find in this book, to help them explore and harness the power of their dreams.

This book is dedicated to those who are curious and ready to delve into the depths of their inner selves. It is for those who wish to learn lessons from their subconscious, gain insights into their own psyche, and uncover truths about themselves and the world around them that they never knew before. Lucid dreaming is not just a nightly escape; it is a journey of self-discovery and personal transformation.

As you turn these pages, you will find comprehensive techniques, practical advice, and inspiring anecdotes to guide you on your path to mastering lucid dreaming. Whether you are a beginner or an experienced dreamer, this guide is designed to help you unlock your inner dreamer and transform your life.

With gratitude,

Violet

Why Lucid Dreaming Matters

Have you ever wished to unlock a hidden realm within your mind, where creativity knows no bounds, and possibilities are endless? Lucid dreaming is your key to this extraordinary world. It is the art of becoming aware that you are dreaming while still in the dream state, granting you the ability to control and shape your dreams. Imagine painting the skies with your thoughts or solving complex problems with the freedom and fluidity that only dreams can offer.

Lucid dreaming is more than just fantastical escapades; it's a powerful tool for real-life transformation. By consciously exploring your dreams, you tap into a deeper well of creativity and insight. This practice can significantly enhance your problem-solving abilities, allowing you to approach challenges with fresh, innovative perspectives. Moreover, lucid dreaming offers a unique path to self-awareness, helping you uncover the hidden facets of your personality and understand what truly drives you.

In this guide, we will delve into the mechanics of lucid dreaming, revealing how it works and how you can harness its potential. You'll learn practical techniques to start practicing lucid dreaming, transforming your nights into a playground of possibilities. Whether you're seeking personal growth, creative inspiration, or simply a thrilling adventure, lucid dreaming is your gateway to a world where your wildest dreams come true.

So, are you ready to step into this mesmerizing realm of exploration and opportunity? Prepare to unlock your inner dreamer and embark on a journey like no other. Welcome to the magic of lucid dreaming!

Chapter 1: The Basics of Lucid Dreaming

Definition and Key Concepts

Welcome to the captivating world of lucid dreaming! Imagine being fully aware that you are dreaming while still in the dream state. That's what lucid dreaming is all about. It's an exhilarating experience where the dreamer realizes that the unfolding events are not real, yet they feel strikingly vivid and genuine. For some, this awareness opens the door to an extraordinary ability to control their dreams, shaping the narrative, characters, and environments like a director crafting a masterpiece. Remarkably, over half of the population has experienced lucid dreaming at least once in their lives.

Lucid dreaming is a fascinating intersection between conscious awareness and the subconscious mind. It's not merely about realizing you're dreaming; it's about harnessing that realization to explore and influence your dream world. The potential benefits are vast, ranging from enhanced creativity and problem-solving skills to profound self-discovery and emotional healing.

History of Lucid Dreaming

Lucid dreaming isn't a modern invention; it's a concept steeped in history. Over 2,000 years ago, the Greek philosopher Aristotle was the first to document the phenomenon in his work "On Dreams." He described moments of awareness within dreams, sparking centuries of fascination and exploration.

Eastern religious traditions, particularly Buddhism, have long valued the awareness of dream states. Tibetan Buddhists practice a form of dream yoga, aiming to use dreams as a path to enlightenment and deeper understanding of the mind.

Despite its ancient roots, scientific exploration of lucid dreaming began in earnest only in the 19th century. The 1960s and 1970s marked a significant breakthrough with the development of the electrooculogram (EOG). This technology allowed researchers to detect specific eye movements signaling consciousness within dreams, providing the first objective evidence that lucid dreaming occurs during REM sleep.

How Lucid Dreams Occur

The science behind lucid dreaming is as intriguing as the experience itself. Neurological and psychological research reveals that lucid dreaming is closely linked to metacognitive abilities—the capacity to observe and regulate our own thought processes. Individuals with heightened self-awareness are more likely to experience lucid dreams.

Technological advancements like the electroencephalogram (EEG) have revolutionized our understanding of brain activity during lucid dreaming. These tools allow scientists to monitor brain waves and physiological markers, offering a detailed glimpse into the brain's inner workings during a lucid dream.

Modern Scientific Research

Current scholarly research continues to expand our understanding of lucid dreaming. Studies have shown that lucid dreaming occurs primarily during REM (Rapid Eye Movement) sleep, a stage of sleep characterized by rapid eye movements, increased brain activity, and vivid dreams. During REM sleep, the brain exhibits activity patterns similar to those during wakefulness, which may explain why lucid dreaming feels so real.

Neuroscientific studies using functional MRI (fMRI) have revealed that specific areas of the brain are active during lucid dreaming, particularly the prefrontal cortex, which is involved in self-awareness and decision-making. This suggests that lucid dreaming is not just a passive state but involves active cognitive processes.

Recent research has also explored the potential therapeutic applications of lucid dreaming. For instance, lucid dreaming therapy (LDT) has been used to help individuals overcome nightmares, PTSD, and other anxiety-related conditions. By becoming aware within their dreams, individuals can confront and alter distressing dream scenarios, leading to reduced symptoms and improved mental health.

Chapter 2: How to Experience a Lucid Dream

Embarking on the journey of lucid dreaming requires dedication and a few key strategies to improve your chances of success. In this chapter, we will explore various methods to help you achieve lucid dreams more frequently and vividly, supported by current scholarly research.

Improving REM Sleep

The foundation of lucid dreaming lies in getting sufficient REM sleep, the stage of sleep where most vivid dreaming occurs. To enhance your REM sleep:

- **Maintain a Regular Sleep Schedule**: Go to bed and wake up at the same time every day, even on weekends. Research shows that consistent sleep patterns can significantly improve sleep quality and REM sleep duration.

- **Create a Relaxing Bedtime Routine**: Avoid screens and stimulating activities before bed. Instead, engage in calming activities like reading a book or taking a warm bath. Blue light from screens can interfere with melatonin production, disrupting your sleep cycle.

- **Avoid Caffeine and Heavy Meals**: Steer clear of caffeine and large meals in the hours leading up to bedtime. Studies have shown that caffeine can delay sleep onset and reduce REM sleep, while heavy meals can cause discomfort and disrupt sleep.

- **Optimize Your Sleep Environment**: Ensure your bedroom is cool, dark, and quiet to promote restful sleep. According to the National Sleep Foundation, a comfortable sleep environment can significantly enhance sleep quality.

Dream Recall Techniques

Improving your ability to recall dreams is crucial for lucid dreaming. Here's how you can enhance your dream recall:

- **Keep a Dream Journal**: Write down your dreams as soon as you wake up. This practice helps you remember more details over time. Research suggests that keeping a dream journal can improve dream recall and increase the likelihood of lucid dreaming.

- **Review Your Dream Journal Regularly**: Re-reading your entries can reinforce your dream recall abilities and increase your awareness of recurring themes or symbols. This reflective practice can help you recognize patterns and triggers for lucid dreaming.

Reality Testing

Reality testing involves regularly questioning whether you are awake or dreaming. This practice can help increase your awareness and improve the chances of becoming lucid in your dreams. Some reality testing techniques include:

- **Finger through Palm Test**: Try pushing your finger through the palm of your other hand. In a dream, your finger might pass through, indicating you are dreaming. This test leverages the peculiar physics of dreams, where physical laws often do not apply.

- **Nose Pinch Test**: Pinch your nose and try to breathe through it. If you can still breathe, you're likely in a dream. This simple test can be very effective due to the distinct physiological responses in dreams.

- **Check Clocks and Texts**: Look at a clock or a piece of text, look away, and then look back. In a dream, the time or text may change or appear distorted. This method exploits the unstable nature of written text and numbers in dreams.

Mnemonic Induction of Lucid Dreams (MILD)

MILD is a popular technique for inducing lucid dreams. It involves using your intention to recognize that you are dreaming. Here's how to practice MILD:

- **Set an Intention**: Before falling asleep, repeat a phrase like "I will realize I'm dreaming" to yourself. This technique is based on prospective memory, the ability to remember to perform a specific action in the future.

- **Visualize Yourself Becoming Lucid**: Imagine a recent dream and picture yourself becoming aware that you are dreaming within that scenario. Visualization strengthens your intention and primes your mind for lucidity.

- **Practice Consistently**: Repeat this process each night to reinforce your intention. Studies have shown that regular practice of MILD can significantly increase the frequency of lucid dreams.

Meditation and Relaxation Techniques

Relaxation and mindfulness practices can significantly enhance your ability to achieve lucid dreams. Incorporate these techniques into your routine:

- **Meditation**: Regular meditation can improve your overall awareness and mindfulness, which can carry over into your dream state. Research indicates that mindfulness meditation can increase dream recall and the likelihood of lucid dreams.

- **Visualization**: Before bed, visualize yourself becoming lucid in a dream. Picture the details vividly and imagine the sensation of becoming aware within the dream. Visualization can strengthen the mental pathways needed for lucid dreaming.
- **Progressive Relaxation**: Practice progressive muscle relaxation to release tension and prepare your mind for sleep. This technique can help you enter a relaxed state conducive to lucid dreaming.

Keeping a Positive Attitude

Maintaining an optimistic mindset is essential for success in lucid dreaming. A positive attitude helps you overcome obstacles and persist in your practice. Remember, each attempt is a learning experience, and even if you don't achieve lucidity every time, you're gaining valuable insights.

Acknowledging the Dream State

Once you become aware that you're dreaming, the next step is to acknowledge and maintain that awareness. Pay attention to your thoughts, emotions, and surroundings within the dream. This mindfulness will help you stay lucid and control the dream more effectively.

Persistence and Open-mindedness

Lucid dreaming is a skill that takes time to develop. Be patient and consistent with your practice, viewing each attempt as an opportunity to learn. Stay open-minded and curious about your dream experiences, allowing your creativity to flourish and uncovering new possibilities within your subconscious mind.

With these strategies, you are well on your way to unlocking your inner dreamer and experiencing the power of lucid dreaming. As you develop your skills and explore your dreams more deeply, it becomes crucial to recognize when you are truly in a lucid dream. In the next chapter, we will delve into the techniques and signs that help you know if your dream is lucid, guiding you further on this exciting journey.

Chapter 3: How to Know if Your Dream is Lucid

Most of the time, during non-lucid dreams, we are unaware that we are dreaming. These dreams often feel remarkably real, even when bizarre or impossible things happen. It's only upon waking that we realize it was just a dream. However, in a lucid dream, the dreamer is aware that they are dreaming and recognizes that the events are not real. This awareness often allows the dreamer to influence or control the dream's course.

Signs of Lucidity

How can you tell if a dream was lucid? Here are some key indicators:

- **Awareness of Dreaming**: You know that you are dreaming and that the events unfolding are not real. This self-awareness distinguishes lucid dreams from non-lucid ones. Awareness within the dream state is a critical component of lucidity.

- **Conscious Decision-Making**: In the dream, you can make deliberate choices about what happens next or how to react to various situations. This level of control and intentionality is a hallmark of lucidity. Studies have shown that the prefrontal cortex, responsible for decision-making and self-awareness, is more active during lucid dreaming.

- **Vivid Details**: Lucid dreams often have strikingly vivid details. You can recall specific colors, shapes, objects, and characters with clarity. The sensory richness of these dreams can be extraordinary. Research in Consciousness and Cognition has highlighted the heightened sensory perception in lucid dreams.

- **Emotional Intensity**: Emotions in lucid dreams can be incredibly intense. Whether it's joy, fear, excitement, or wonder, the feelings you experience are often amplified, adding to the vividness of the dream. Studies suggest that the amygdala, which processes emotions, is highly active during these dreams.

- **Control over the Dream Environment**: You may have the ability to manipulate the dream setting or characters. For instance, you might find yourself flying, moving objects with your mind, or altering the dream's landscape. A study in Nature Neuroscience found that lucid dreamers often report a higher degree of control within their dreams.

- **Clear Memory Upon Waking:** Lucid dreams are typically remembered more clearly than non-lucid ones. You can recall the sequence of events, the decisions you made, and the emotions you felt with great detail. The Journal of Sleep Research notes that lucid dreams tend to be more memorable due to their heightened awareness and sensory experiences.

If any of these signs sound familiar, you may have already experienced a lucid dream. Recognizing these indicators is the first step toward becoming more proficient in lucid dreaming.

Maintaining Lucidity

Once you realize you are dreaming, maintaining that lucidity can be challenging. Here are some techniques to help you stay lucid:

- **Stay Calm:** The excitement of realizing you're dreaming can sometimes wake you up. Practice staying calm and grounded to prolong the dream. Research indicates that emotional regulation techniques can help maintain lucidity.
- **Engage Your Senses:** Focus on the sensory details of the dream, such as touching objects or observing the environment closely. This can help stabilize the

dream and maintain lucidity. Sensory engagement has been shown to anchor dreamers in the dream state.

- **Use Affirmations**: Repeating phrases like "I am aware that I am dreaming" can reinforce your lucidity and keep you focused. Affirmations can act as mental cues to remind you of your dream state.

- **Practice Reality Checks**: Even within the dream, continue performing reality checks to reaffirm that you are dreaming. This can help sustain your awareness. Reality checks are effective because they create a habit of questioning reality, which carries over into dreams.

- **Set Goals**: Before going to sleep, set specific goals for what you want to do in your lucid dream. Having a clear purpose can keep you engaged and prolong the lucid state. Goal-setting in dreams can increase motivation and focus.

Techniques Supported by Current Research

- **Neurofeedback**: Emerging studies suggest that neurofeedback training can enhance your ability to achieve and maintain lucid dreams by increasing your awareness of brainwave patterns associated with lucidity.

- **Targeted Memory Reactivation (TMR):** This technique involves exposing yourself to specific cues (such as sounds) during REM sleep to trigger lucidity. Research has shown promising results, with increased instances of lucid dreaming in participants who used TMR.

By mastering these techniques and staying informed about the latest research, you can enhance your ability to remain lucid and fully explore the possibilities within your dreams. Recognizing and maintaining lucidity in your dreams opens up a world of opportunities for creativity, problem-solving, and personal growth.

As you develop your skills and explore your dreams more deeply, it's essential to understand how to apply them effectively. In the next chapter, we will delve into the practical applications of lucid dreaming, helping you unlock its full potential for creativity, problem-solving, and personal growth. Your journey into the depths of your subconscious has just begun. Good luck on your path to mastering lucid dreaming!

Chapter 4: Uses of Lucid Dreaming

Lucid dreaming, with its immersive and vivid experiences, offers a unique opportunity to explore the inner workings of our minds with heightened awareness. Some researchers have described it as "the ultimate form of immersive experience," providing a safe, fantastical world where anything becomes possible. The extraordinary sensory and emotional experiences associated with lucid dreaming make it highly appealing. Beyond its allure as a unique experience, lucid dreaming holds real-world applications that can significantly benefit various aspects of our lives.

Enhanced Creativity

Imagine having a limitless playground for your imagination every night. Lucid dreaming allows you to experiment creatively and explore new ideas without the constraints of reality. Dreamers have the ability to construct or invent anything, experiencing and exploring things they might not be able to in daily life. Studies have shown that lucid dreamers often perform better on creativity tests and feel more inspired and creative after their experiences. The dream world, with its magical qualities and lack of physical boundaries, allows for boundless creativity, offering new perspectives and stimulating inner creativity that can be applied in waking life. Just think of it as your own personal brainstorming session, where the only limit is your imagination.

Therapeutic Benefits

Fewer Nightmares

For those plagued by nightmares, lucid dreaming can be a game-changer. Bad dreams can disrupt sleep and negatively impact your overall well-being. By becoming aware within their dreams, lucid dreamers can control or change the course of their nightmares, transforming them into more calming or pleasant experiences. This ability to influence dreams can reduce the frequency and intensity of nightmares, contributing to better sleep and overall well-being. Imagine turning a terrifying chase into a serene walk through a beautiful garden – the power is in your hands.

Improved Mental Health and Well-being

Lucid dreaming offers a unique avenue for addressing mental health issues. Imagine being able to confront and overcome your fears within the safety of a dream. This can be particularly beneficial for those struggling with anxiety or post-traumatic stress disorder (PTSD). Lucid dreaming can serve as a self-therapeutic tool, enabling individuals to symbolically address and resolve challenging issues in a safe, controlled environment. By practicing relaxation and control in dream scenarios, dreamers can reduce anxiety and improve their mental health and well-being. It's like having your own therapy session while you sleep.

Personal Growth

Lucid dreaming offers profound opportunities for personal growth. By accessing the subconscious mind, individuals can gain deeper insights into themselves and their behavior. This heightened self-awareness can help break free from limiting beliefs or emotional blocks, fostering mindfulness and a better understanding of one's waking life. Lucid dreams can provide unexpected wisdom and clarity on situations, aiding in personal development and growth. Think of it as a nightly journey of self-discovery, where you can learn more about who you are and what drives you.

Practical Applications

Improved Problem-Solving Skills

Lucid dreamers are more conscious of their thoughts, emotions, and behavior in the dreamscape, leading to improved mental clarity and problem-solving skills. By recognizing patterns that may be hidden in normal dreams, lucid dreamers can gain valuable insights into their minds and develop creative solutions to problems. This enhanced mental clarity can translate into better decision-making and problem-solving abilities in waking life. It's like having a mental workshop where you can tinker with ideas and solutions without any real-world consequences.

Enhanced Self-Awareness

The awareness cultivated through lucid dreaming extends beyond the dream state, leading to improved self-awareness and a general understanding of life. Dreamers can explore their subconscious, uncovering insights and clarity that can help resolve real-life issues. This deeper connection to the subconscious mind can lead to more mindful living and a better grasp of one's thoughts and emotions. Imagine being more in tune with yourself, understanding your motivations and behaviors on a deeper level.

New Perspectives on Life

Lucid dreaming can inspire new perspectives and stimulate inner creativity that can be used in everyday life. The dream world, with its limitless possibilities, allows individuals to explore new hobbies, expand existing ones, and devise creative solutions to problems. Lucid dreaming opens up opportunities for innovation and creative thinking, providing access to parts of the psyche that might otherwise remain untapped. It's like having a creative muse that visits you every night, helping you think outside the box and see the world in new ways.

Improved Interpersonal Relationships

Finally, lucid dreaming can enhance interpersonal relationships by offering insights into one's behavior and interactions with others. Dreamers can explore complex relationships and practice communication skills or confront difficult conversations in a safe, judgment-free space. By becoming aware of behavior patterns during dreams, individuals can gain valuable insights into how they interact with family, friends, co-workers, and strangers, ultimately improving their real-life relationships. It's like having a rehearsal space where you can work through social challenges and improve your interactions with others.

With these varied and profound applications, lucid dreaming is more than just an extraordinary experience; it is a powerful tool for creativity, therapy, personal growth, and practical problem-solving. However, as with any powerful tool, it's essential to understand its potential pitfalls. In the next chapter, we'll delve into the mental health considerations, potential negative effects on sleep quality, and managing expectations regarding lucid dreaming. Your exploration of lucid dreaming is just beginning, and it's important to be mindful of both its wonders and its challenges as you continue this fascinating journey.

Chapter 5: Potential Pitfalls of Lucid Dreaming

While lucid dreaming offers a gateway to incredible experiences, creativity, and self-exploration, it's essential to be aware of potential pitfalls. Understanding these risks will help you navigate your lucid dreaming journey safely and effectively, ensuring that you can fully enjoy the benefits while mitigating any negative effects.

Mental Health Considerations

Lucid dreaming can have both positive and negative impacts on mental health. While it can be therapeutic and provide a sense of control, several studies suggest potential drawbacks.

Negative Mental Health Impacts

Some research indicates that vivid lucid dreams might be linked to increased psychopathological symptoms. For instance, frequent lucid dreamers may have a higher risk of experiencing depression, dissociation, and other mental health issues. A study published in Frontiers in Psychology suggests that long-term engagement in lucid dreaming practices could potentially lead to these negative outcomes. Therefore, it's crucial to approach lucid dreaming with caution, especially if you have a history of mental health concerns.

Increased Anxiety or Panic

The intense nature of controlling your dreams can sometimes be overwhelming, particularly if you're unprepared. Lucid dreams often bring repressed emotions to the surface, which can increase anxiety or even trigger panic attacks. To mitigate these effects, practice mindfulness techniques and relaxation exercises before attempting lucid dreaming. Staying calm and in control is essential to having a positive experience.

Sleep Quality

Lucid dreaming can sometimes disrupt your sleep, leading to poorer sleep quality and overall well-being.

Sleep Interruptions

Lucid dreams are often intense and emotionally charged, which can disturb your sleep. Additionally, some induction techniques, like the Mnemonic Induction of Lucid Dreams (MILD) approach, involve waking up in the middle of the night and staying awake for a period before returning to sleep. While these methods can enhance the likelihood of lucid dreaming, they can also negatively impact sleep duration and quality. Poor sleep can, in turn, affect your mental health and general well-being.

Managing Expectations

Understanding that not all lucid dreaming experiences will be positive is crucial for maintaining a healthy approach to this practice.

Handling Bad Dreams

Lucid dreaming can sometimes lead to nightmares or unsettling experiences. Although it's often seen as an opportunity to control your dreams, the subconscious mind can still create frightening scenarios. Having a plan for handling nightmares, such as repeating calming affirmations or focusing on pleasant memories, can help you manage these situations effectively.

The Role of Personality

Certain personality traits may influence your experience with lucid dreaming.

Personality and Lucid Dreaming

Research suggests a connection between certain psychological qualities and the likelihood of experiencing lucid dreams. For instance, individuals with a strong sense of internal control and higher scores on creativity and cognitive tests are more likely to have lucid dreams. A slight association has also been found between lucid dreaming and the personality trait of openness to experience. Understanding your personality can help you gauge how you might respond to lucid dreaming practices.

Creating a Balanced Approach

To ensure a safe and enjoyable lucid dreaming experience, it's important to take a balanced approach that considers your mental health, personality type, and lifestyle.

Tips for a Positive Experience

1. **Prioritize Sleep**: Ensure you get adequate sleep to be well-rested before attempting lucid dreaming. Quality sleep lays the foundation for a more stable and controllable dream environment.
2. **Practice Relaxation**: Engage in relaxation exercises before bed to help you enter a calm state conducive to positive dreaming experiences. Techniques such as progressive muscle relaxation or deep breathing can be particularly effective.
3. **Develop Coping Strategies**: Prepare calming techniques to use if you encounter nightmares or

frightening dream scenarios. This might include mentally rehearsing positive affirmations or visualizing a safe, comforting space within your dream.

By being aware of these potential risks and taking appropriate measures, you can enjoy the benefits of lucid dreaming while minimizing the drawbacks. With mindful preparation and a balanced approach, you can safely explore the powerful potential of lucid dreaming and unlock your inner dreamer.

Next Steps

Your journey into the depths of your subconscious has just begun. In the next chapter, we'll delve into advanced techniques for lucid dreaming, exploring sophisticated methods and tools to deepen your practice and enhance your dream experiences. These techniques will help you maintain lucidity and maximize the benefits of your lucid dreams. Prepare to elevate your lucid dreaming practice and continue expanding your dreaming horizons.

Chapter 6: Advanced Techniques for Lucid Dreaming

As you deepen your practice of lucid dreaming, you may find yourself seeking more advanced techniques to enhance and expand your experiences. This chapter will introduce you to several sophisticated methods and tools that can help you achieve and maintain lucidity in your dreams.

Wake-Induced Lucid Dreaming (WILD)

Wake-Induced Lucid Dreaming (WILD) is one of the most powerful techniques for inducing lucid dreams. This method involves transitioning directly from a waking state into a lucid dream, maintaining consciousness throughout the process. WILD can lead to highly vivid and controllable lucid dreams, but it requires practice and patience to master.

How to Practice WILD

1. **Preparation**: Wake yourself up after 4 to 6 hours of sleep. Get out of bed and stay awake for anywhere between a few minutes to an hour before going back to bed. It's preferable to engage in activities related to lucid dreaming during this time, such as reading about it or writing in your dream journal.

2. **Relaxation**: Go back to bed and lie absolutely still, as if your body is melting into the mattress. Focus on relaxing each part of your body, starting from your toes and working your way up to your head. Deep breathing can help you achieve a calm and relaxed state.

3. **Mental Focus**: Silence your inner monologue and focus your mind on a single point or imagine a simple scene. This could be anything from a spinning object to a serene landscape. The goal is to keep your mind engaged and prevent it from drifting into unconsciousness.

4. **Hypnagogic State**: As you start to fall asleep, you will enter the hypnagogic state—a transitional phase between wakefulness and sleep characterized by vivid imagery and sensations. Stay focused on your mental image and observe the hypnagogic imagery without becoming too involved.

5. **Entering the Dream**: As the hypnagogic state deepens, you will begin to feel a sense of detachment from your physical body. You may experience sleep

paralysis, a natural protection mechanism that stops you from acting out your dreams. Relax and allow the dream scene to form. Often, the dream environment will start as a familiar place, such as your bedroom, but you can eventually transport yourself to other dreamscapes.

6. **Staying Lucid**: Engage your senses by touching objects, observing your surroundings, and performing reality checks to stabilize and maintain lucidity. Practice makes it increasingly easier to cross over to dreamland fully lucid.

Variations of WILD

1. **Hypnagogic Drop-In**: After waking up and writing down your dreams, set your intent to gain lucidity and allow yourself to drift back into sleep. Focus on the hypnagogic imagery, gently floating through it until the dreamscape forms. Maintain a delicate vigilance without blacking out.

2. **Body and Breath Awareness**: Focus on the sensations in your body and the breath flowing through it as you enter the hypnagogic state. Systematically scan your awareness through your body

or simply allow bodily sensations to attract your attention. This technique is suitable for those with good body awareness, such as dancers or yoga practitioners.

3. **Counting Sleep**: Combine counting with a repeated question to maintain awareness as you transition from wakefulness into a dream. For example, count "One: Am I dreaming? Two: Am I dreaming?" and so on. The aim is to reach a point where you can answer, "Yes, I'm dreaming! I'm lucid!" as you find yourself fully conscious within the dream.

Lucid Dreaming Supplements

Certain supplements are believed to enhance the likelihood and intensity of lucid dreams. These supplements work by affecting neurotransmitter levels and sleep cycles, making it easier to achieve and maintain lucidity. Here are some commonly used supplements, along with information on their safety and effectiveness:

Common Supplements

1. **Galantamine**: Galantamine is a natural alkaloid that inhibits the breakdown of acetylcholine, a neurotransmitter associated with REM sleep and

dreaming. Research suggests that galantamine can significantly increase the frequency and vividness of lucid dreams. However, it should be used with caution, as it can cause side effects such as nausea and gastrointestinal discomfort.

2. **Choline**: Choline is a precursor to acetylcholine and is often used in conjunction with galantamine. It helps enhance the effects of galantamine and promotes vivid dreaming. Choline supplements are generally considered safe when taken in appropriate doses.

3. **Melatonin**: Melatonin is a hormone that regulates sleep-wake cycles. Low doses of melatonin can help improve sleep quality and promote more vivid dreams. However, high doses can disrupt sleep patterns, so it's important to use it cautiously.

4. **5-HTP (5-Hydroxytryptophan)**: 5-HTP is a precursor to serotonin, a neurotransmitter that influences mood and sleep. It can enhance dream vividness and recall, but it may also lead to more intense and sometimes disturbing dreams.

Safety and Effectiveness

While these supplements can enhance lucid dreaming, it's crucial to approach them with caution. Always consult with a healthcare professional before starting any supplement regimen, especially if you have underlying health conditions or are taking other medications. Additionally, it's important to start with low doses to assess your body's response and avoid potential side effects.

Technological Aids

In the digital age, various devices and apps have been developed to assist with lucid dreaming. These technological aids can help you track your sleep patterns, induce lucid dreams, and maintain awareness during sleep.

Devices

1. **Lucid Dream Masks**: These masks are equipped with LED lights and sensors that detect when you enter REM sleep. The lights flash gently, signaling you that you are dreaming without waking you up. Examples include the NovaDreamer and the Remee mask.

2. **EEG Headbands**: EEG headbands monitor brainwave activity and can help identify when you are in a dream state. They can provide audio or visual

cues to help you become aware that you are dreaming. The Muse headband is a popular option for this purpose.

Apps

1. **Lucidity Apps**: Apps like Awoken and Lucid Dreamer offer reality check reminders, dream journals, and induction techniques to support your lucid dreaming practice. They can help you stay consistent with your practice and provide valuable insights into your dream patterns.

2. **Sleep Tracking Apps**: Apps such as Sleep Cycle and Pillow analyze your sleep patterns and provide data on your REM cycles. This information can help you identify the best times for practicing lucid dream induction techniques.

By incorporating advanced techniques, supplements, and technological aids into your lucid dreaming practice, you can enhance your ability to achieve and maintain lucidity in your dreams. These tools offer exciting opportunities to explore the depths of your subconscious mind and unlock new levels of creativity, problem-solving, and personal growth.

As you continue to refine your skills and experiment with these methods, you may find that your lucid dreams become more vivid, frequent, and meaningful. In the next chapter, we will delve into case studies and research on lucid dreaming, providing real-world examples and scientific insights to further inspire and guide your practice. Then, we will explore how to integrate lucid dreaming into your daily life, ensuring it complements rather than disrupts your waking world.

Chapter 7: Case Studies and Research

Lucid dreaming has fascinated humans for centuries, but only in recent decades has it gained significant scientific recognition. This chapter explores key studies on lucid dreaming, offering insights from historical and modern research and examining the technological advancements that have enhanced our understanding of this intriguing phenomenon.

Historical and Modern Research

Early Research

The scientific exploration of lucid dreaming began in earnest in the mid-20th century. Celia Green's pioneering research in 1968 laid the groundwork for our understanding of lucid dreams. She discovered that lucid dreams are connected to REM (Rapid Eye Movement) sleep and was the first to link lucid dreams and false awakenings. Her work illuminated the basic mechanics of lucid dreaming, providing a foundation for future studies.

In 1975, Keith Hearne conducted groundbreaking experiments with a skilled lucid dreamer. Using an electrooculogram (EOG) to track eye movements, Hearne aimed to enable the dreamer to communicate with the waking world directly from their dreams. The findings, published in a well-known journal, sparked further scientific curiosity and led to more extensive research on lucid dreaming.

Advances in the 1980s

The 1980s saw significant contributions from Stephen LaBerge, a pioneer in lucid dreaming research. LaBerge's studies demonstrated that time perception in lucid dreams is similar to that in waking life. He also found that different activities in lucid dreams activate various brain hemispheres. His work greatly advanced our understanding of the mechanisms behind lucid dreaming and how to optimize the experience.

Scientific Insights

Brain Activity during Lucid Dreaming

Recent research has provided fascinating insights into the brain's activity during lucid dreaming. In 2007, Ursula Voss and her colleagues published a study in the Journal of Consciousness Studies, revealing that lucid dreamers exhibit increased gamma wave activity during REM sleep. Gamma waves are associated with higher levels of consciousness and attention. The study also used Transcranial Magnetic Stimulation (TMS), a non-invasive method that uses magnetic fields to stimulate brain cells, to induce lucid dreams. This research highlighted the potential of TMS to enhance our understanding of lucid dreaming.

Neurological Research

Further studies have explored the neurological aspects of lucid dreaming. Research has shown that the size of the anterior prefrontal cortex is linked to the ability to experience lucid dreams. Functional MRI (fMRI) scans revealed that lucid dreamers have increased activity in the prefrontal cortex, which is involved in higher-order thinking, self-reflection, and planning. Elisa Filevich at the Max Planck Institute for Human Development noted that "self-reflection in everyday life is more pronounced in persons who can easily control their dreams," suggesting that frequent lucid dreamers may have superior introspection and planning skills.

Dr. Daniel Erlacher from the University of Bern conducted studies indicating that lucid dreamers show enhanced frontal brain activity. This area is crucial for metacognitive processes, making sense that the frontal lobe would be connected to the characteristics of lucid dreams. The dorsolateral prefrontal cortex (DLPFC), responsible for abstract thinking and decision-making, is also impacted by lucid dreaming. This brain region is linked to higher-order cognition, executive function, and working memory and may play a significant role in the sensation of self-consciousness or meta-awareness during lucid dreams.

These findings suggest a strong link between lucid dreaming and increased brain activity in areas associated with higher-order thinking, self-awareness, and visuospatial processing. Lucid dreaming might also enhance cognitive abilities and improve sleep quality, though further research is needed to confirm these benefits.

Technological Advances in Research

Technological advancements have revolutionized the study of lucid dreaming, providing tools that allow for more precise and controlled experiments. Devices such as EEG headbands and lucid dream masks have enabled researchers to monitor brainwave activity and provide cues to help dreamers become aware that they are dreaming. These tools have made it easier to study lucid dreaming in controlled settings and have contributed significantly to our understanding of the phenomenon.

The scientific study of lucid dreaming has come a long way since its early days, with modern research and technological advancements significantly enhancing our understanding of this fascinating phenomenon. The insights gained from these studies deepen our knowledge of the brain and consciousness and open up exciting possibilities for practical applications in creativity, therapy, and personal growth.

As you develop your skills and explore your dreams more deeply, it's essential to understand how to apply them effectively. In the next chapter, we will explore how to integrate lucid dreaming into your daily life, ensuring it complements rather than disrupts your waking world. By building a supportive routine and understanding the long-term benefits, you can fully harness the power of lucid dreaming.

Chapter 8: Integrating Lucid Dreaming into Your Life

Lucid dreaming offers a unique opportunity to explore your subconscious mind, enhance creativity, and improve personal growth. To fully benefit from lucid dreaming, it is essential to integrate it seamlessly into your daily life. This chapter will guide you on how to create a routine that supports lucid dreaming, balance dream practices with your waking life, and understand the long-term advantages of regular lucid dreaming.

Building a Routine

Creating a supportive routine for lucid dreaming involves incorporating specific habits and techniques into your daily life. Consistency and dedication are key to fostering an environment conducive to lucid dreaming.

Establish a Consistent Sleep Schedule

- **Regular Bedtime and Wake Time:** Go to bed and wake up at the same time every day, including weekends. This helps regulate your body's internal clock and ensures you get adequate REM sleep, where lucid dreaming occurs.

- **Pre-Sleep Rituals**: Develop calming pre-sleep rituals such as reading, meditating, or taking a warm bath. Avoid screens and stimulating activities at least an hour before bed to enhance sleep quality.

Keep a Dream Journal

- **Recording Dreams**: Keep a journal by your bedside and write down your dreams as soon as you wake up. Note details, emotions, and any patterns you observe. This practice enhances dream recall and increases the likelihood of becoming lucid in future dreams.
- **Reviewing Entries**: Regularly review your dream journal entries. Look for recurring themes or symbols that might help you recognize when you are dreaming.

Perform Reality Checks

- **Daily Practice**: Incorporate reality checks into your daily routine. Techniques like the finger-through-palm test or the nose pinch test can help you question your reality and increase your awareness during dreams.
- **Mindful Moments**: Throughout the day, pause and ask yourself if you are dreaming. This habit can carry

over into your dream state, making it easier to recognize when you are dreaming.

Use Induction Techniques

- **Mnemonic Induction of Lucid Dreams (MILD):** Before falling asleep, repeat a phrase like "I will realize I'm dreaming" to yourself. Visualize yourself becoming lucid in a recent dream.

- **Wake-Back-to-Bed (WBTB):** Set an alarm to wake up after 4-6 hours of sleep. Stay awake for 15-60 minutes, engaging in a quiet activity like reading about lucid dreaming, then go back to sleep with the intention of becoming lucid.

Balancing Dream and Reality

While lucid dreaming offers numerous benefits, it's crucial to ensure that it complements rather than disrupts your waking life. Here are strategies to maintain a healthy balance:

Prioritize Quality Sleep

- **Avoid Sleep Disruptions:** While techniques like WBTB are effective, overusing them can lead to fragmented sleep. Ensure you get sufficient uninterrupted sleep to maintain overall health and well-being.

- **Healthy Sleep Hygiene**: Maintain good sleep hygiene by creating a sleep-friendly environment—cool, dark, and quiet—and avoiding caffeine or heavy meals before bedtime.

Set Boundaries

1. **Time Management**: Allocate specific times for lucid dreaming practices, such as during weekends or vacations, to avoid interference with your daily responsibilities.
2. **Mindfulness Practices**: Engage in mindfulness or meditation practices to help ground yourself in the present moment and balance your dream experiences with reality.

Long-Term Benefits

Integrating lucid dreaming into your life can offer lasting benefits that extend beyond the dream state. Here are some of the advantages you can expect:

Enhanced Creativity and Problem-Solving

- **Creative Exploration**: Lucid dreaming allows you to explore new ideas and solutions in a limitless environment. This can enhance your creativity and provide innovative solutions to real-world problems.
- **Cognitive Flexibility**: Regular lucid dreaming practice can improve your cognitive flexibility, helping you think more creatively and adaptively in waking life.

Emotional and Psychological Growth

- **Emotional Healing**: Lucid dreaming provides a safe space to confront and resolve emotional issues, leading to improved mental health and emotional well-being.
- **Self-Discovery**: By exploring your subconscious mind, you can gain deeper insights into your behavior, motivations, and beliefs, fostering personal growth and self-awareness.

Improved Sleep Quality

- **Restful Sleep**: Contrary to concerns about sleep disruption, many lucid dreamers report improved sleep quality and more restful sleep. Lucid dreaming can make your sleep experience more enjoyable and rejuvenating.

- **Dream Control:** Learning to control your dreams can reduce the frequency of nightmares and improve overall sleep satisfaction.

Mindfulness and Awareness

- **Increased Mindfulness:** The practices involved in lucid dreaming, such as reality checks and mindfulness, can enhance your overall awareness and presence in daily life.
- **Enhanced Focus:** Developing the skill to stay lucid in dreams can improve your ability to focus and maintain concentration in waking life.

Conclusion

Lucid dreaming is a profound journey of self-discovery, creativity, and personal growth. Embrace this journey with curiosity and an open mind. Each dream is an opportunity to explore the depths of your subconscious and uncover new aspects of yourself. Stay dedicated to your practice, and remember that every step, whether a small insight or a grand revelation, contributes to your growth.

The future of lucid dreaming research holds exciting possibilities. As scientific understanding of the brain and consciousness expands, new techniques and technologies will continue to enhance our ability to explore and harness the power of lucid dreams. Stay informed about the latest developments and be open to integrating new methods into your practice.

In your personal practice, continue to set goals, experiment with different techniques, and reflect on your experiences. Lucid dreaming is a dynamic and evolving practice, and your journey will evolve as you do. Keep an open heart and mind, and let your inner dreamer guide you to new heights of creativity, healing, and self-awareness.

By fully integrating lucid dreaming into your life, you can unlock its full potential and experience the profound benefits it offers. May your dreams be vivid, your awareness sharp, and your journey ever fascinating.